Table of Contents

PREVIEW

The colonoscopy is performed by a doctor experienced in the procedure and lasts approximately 30-60 minutes. Medications will be given into your vein to make you feel relaxed and drowsy. You will be asked to lie on your left side on the examining table. During a colonoscopy, the doctor uses a colonoscope, a long, flexible, tubular instrument about 1/2-inch in diameter that transmits an image of the lining of the colon so the doctor can examine it for any abnormalities. The colonoscope is inserted through the rectum and advanced to the other end of the large intestine.

ou may feel mild cramping during the procedure. You can reduce the cramping by taking several slow, deep breaths during the procedure. When the doctor has finished, the colonoscope is slowly withdrawn while the lining of your bowel is carefully examined.

During the colonoscopy, if the doctor sees something that may be abnormal, small amounts of tissue can be removed for analysis (called a biopsy), and abnormal growths, or polyps, can be identified and removed. In many cases, colonoscopy allows accurate diagnosis and treatment without the need for a major operation.

COLONOSCOPY DIET RECIPES

BREAKFAST

1. Potato Broccoli Mini Frittatas
Prep-Time: 30 Minutes

Cook Time: 1 hour

Total Time: 1 hour 30 minutes

Servings: 12

Ingredients

- 1½ cups sliced mushrooms (4 oz.)
- 1¼ cups chopped red potatoes (6 oz.)
- ½ cup chopped red bell pepper
- ¼ cup chopped red onion
- 4 cups frozen broccoli florets, thawed and coarsely chopped
- 1½ cups unsweetened, unflavored plant milk, such as almond, soy, cashew, or rice
- 2 tablespoons flaxseed meal
- 1 cup chickpea flour
- 2 tablespoons nutritional yeast
- 1 teaspoon baking powder
- 1 teaspoon dried dill weed
- ¼ teaspoon ground turmeric

- Freshly ground black pepper, to taste
- Chopped fresh herbs, such as chives, tarragon, or parsley (optional)

Instructions

1. Preheat oven to 350°F. Line twelve 2½-inch muffin cups with foil bake cups.

2. In a large skillet cook mushrooms, potatoes, bell pepper, and onion over medium 10 minutes or until tender, stirring occasionally and adding water, 1 to 2 Tbsp. at a time, as needed to prevent sticking. Stir in broccoli.

3. Meanwhile, in a medium bowl stir together milk and flaxseed meal; let stand 5 minutes.

4. Stir vegetable mixture and the next five ingredients (through turmeric) into milk mixture. Spoon about ⅓ cup into each muffin cup.

5. Bake 25 minutes or until center seems set. Let stand in muffin cups on a wire rack 5 minutes. Remove from cups. Serve warm. Season with black pepper and sprinkle with fresh herbs, if using.

2. Muffin Tin Mini Tostadas

Prep-Time: 20 Minutes

Cook Time: 40 Minutes

Total Time: 1 hour

Makes 12 Tostadas

Ingredients

- ½ cup chopped green or red bell pepper
- ¼ cup chopped onion
- 1½ cups cooked ½-inch cubes sweet potato
- ½ of a 15-oz. can no-salt-added black beans, rinsed and drained (¾ cup)
- 12 6-inch corn tortillas, each cut into 6 wedges
- ¾ cup chickpea flour
- 1 tablespoon nutritional yeast
- ¾ teaspoon baking powder
- ¾ teaspoon ground cumin
- ½ teaspoon chipotle chile powder
- ½ teaspoon sea salt
- ½ teaspoon freshly ground black pepper
- 1¼ cups unsweetened, unflavored plant milk, such as almond, soy, cashew, or rice
- 1 cup refrigerated fresh salsa
- Fresh cilantro leaves for garnish (optional)

Instructions

1. Preheat oven to 350°F. Line twelve 2½-inch muffin cups with foil bake cups. In a medium skillet cook bell pepper and onion over medium 3 to 4 minutes or until just tender, stirring occasionally and adding water, 1 to 2 tsp. at a time, as needed to prevent sticking. Remove from heat and stir in sweet potato and black beans.

2. Arrange six tortilla wedges in each prepared muffin cup with curved edges at bottom and points up. (Each should look like a crown.) Spoon about ¼ cup bean mixture into each cup. In a medium bowl stir together the next seven ingredients (through black pepper). Gradually whisk in milk until smooth. Spoon about 2 Tbsp. batter over bean mixture in each cup.

3. Bake 20 to 25 minutes or until filling is set. Carefully remove cups. Top with fresh salsa and cilantro (if desired), and serve immediately.

3. Sweet Potato, Pear, and Blueberry Flatbreads

Prep-Time: 30 Minutes

Cook Time: 30 Minutes

Total Time: 1 hour

Servings: 4

Ingredients

Cornmeal, for dusting:

- 1 recipe Homemade Oil-Free Pizza Dough
- 1 cup cubed peeled sweet potato
- Sea salt and freshly ground black pepper, to taste
- 1 fresh pear, quartered and cored
- ¾ cup fresh blueberries
- 2 tablespoons chopped toasted walnuts
- 4 teaspoons pure maple syrup
- Ground cinnamon

Instructions

1. Preheat oven to 400°F. Lightly sprinkle a large baking sheet with cornmeal.

2. Divide dough into four portions. On a lightly floured surface, roll portions into 7- to 8-inch circles or 10×5-inch ovals. Transfer flatbreads to prepared pan. Bake

10 to 13 minutes or until lightly browned and set (flatbreads may puff). Let cool.

3. In a small saucepan combine sweet potato and enough water to cover. Bring to boiling; reduce heat. Cover and simmer about 10 minutes or until tender. Drain and return to saucepan. Mash with a fork. Season with salt and pepper.

4. Meanwhile, heat a grill pan over medium-high. Cook pear quarters about 3 minutes per cut side or until tender and light grill marks appear. Thinly slice quarters lengthwise.

5. Spread sweet potato on flatbreads. Top with pear slices, blueberries, and walnuts. Drizzle with maple syrup and sprinkle with cinnamon.

4. Roasted Vegetable Breakfast Hash

Prep-Time: 30 Minutes

Cook Time: 15 Minutes

Total Time: 45 minutes

Servings: 9

Ingredients

- ½ of a 12- to 14-oz. pkg. extra-firm light silken tofu
- 2 tablespoons coarse-ground mustard
- 1 tablespoon lemon juice
- 2 teaspoons pure maple syrup
- 1 teaspoon smoked paprika
- 3 medium red potatoes, cut into ½-inch cubes (1 lb.)
- 2 medium sweet potatoes, cut into ½-inch cubes (1 lb.)
- 1 medium onion, coarsely chopped
- 2 carrots, cut into ½-inch cubes
- 2 parsnips, peeled and cut into ½-inch cubes
- 2 medium beets, peeled and cut into ½-inch cubes
- 8 oz. Brussels sprouts, quartered (2 cups)
- Sea salt and freshly ground black pepper, to taste
- Chopped fresh thyme (optional)

Instructions

1. Preheat oven to 400°F. Line two rimmed baking sheets with parchment paper or silicone baking mats. For mustard sauce, in a small food processor or blender combine tofu, mustard, lemon juice, and maple syrup. Cover and process until very smooth. Place 2 tablespoons sauce in a small bowl with 2 tablespoons water and the paprika. Reserve remaining mustard sauce.

2. In a large bowl combine the next five ingredients (through parsnips). Drizzle with most of the diluted paprika sauce. Place in prepared baking sheets, leaving an area for beets. Place beets in the same bowl and toss with remaining paprika sauce; place in baking sheet. Roast vegetables 20 minutes.

3. Sprinkle Brussels sprouts over vegetables in baking sheets, stirring to mix. Roast 20 to 30 minutes more or until all vegetables are tender and starting to brown.

4. In a large serving bowl combine all vegetables. Add ¼ cup water to the reserved mustard sauce and drizzle over vegetables. Season with salt and pepper.

5. Serve hash topped with fresh thyme, if desired. Cool any leftovers and refrigerate in an airtight container up to 3 days.

5. Tortilla Española with Potatoes and Red Peppers

Prep-Time: 40 Minutes

Cook Time: 1 hour

Total Time: 1 hour 40 minutes

Servings: 10

Ingredients

- 2 lb. Yukon gold potatoes, scrubbed and thinly sliced (8 cups)
- 7 oz. extra-firm tofu, drained and patted dry
- ¼ cup + 2 tablespoons aquafaba (liquid from canned chickpeas)
- 2 tablespoons unbleached all-purpose flour or whole wheat flour
- 1 tablespoon chickpea flour
- ⅛ teaspoon ground turmeric
- 2 yellow onions, chopped (2 cups)
- 2 cloves garlic, minced
- ½ cup chopped jarred roasted red bell peppers
- 3 tablespoons finely chopped fresh parsley
- ½ teaspoon black salt or sea salt
- Freshly ground black pepper, to taste

Instructions

1. Preheat oven to 425°F. Place potato pieces in a steamer basket in a large saucepan. Add water to saucepan to just below basket. Bring to boiling. Steam, covered, about 15 minutes or until tender. Transfer to a large bowl.

2. Finely crumble tofu and place in a bowl. Add the next four ingredients (through turmeric); stir to combine.

3. In a large nonstick ovenproof skillet combine onions, garlic, and ¼ cup water. Cook over medium 10 minutes, stirring occasionally and adding water, 1 to 2 Tbsp. at a time, as needed to prevent sticking. Add the remaining ingredients. Cook 2 minutes more to meld flavors. Add potatoes and tofu mixture; mix well.

4. Bake about 30 minutes or until tortilla is golden. Cool tortilla in skillet on a wire rack 10 minutes. Invert a dinner plate over skillet. Holding the plate and skillet together, quickly flip over to invert tortilla onto the plate. Remove skillet. Sprinkle tortilla with additional parsley. Serve warm or at room temperature.

6. Berry-Licious Overnight Oatmeal

Prep-Time: 15 Minutes

Cook Time: 15 minutes

Total Time: 30 minutes

Servings: 4

Ingredients

Overnight Oats:

- 1 cup dry steel-cut oats
- 8 to 10 medium dates, pitted
- ½ teaspoon pure vanilla extract

Sauce:

- 2 cups fresh or frozen strawberries, chopped into large pieces
- 1 cup fresh or frozen raspberries

Toppings

- 1 banana, peeled and sliced
- 1 kiwi, peeled and sliced
- ½ cup fresh blueberries
- ½ tablespoon raisins
- 2 tablespoons sliced almonds
- 1 tablespoon pumpkin seeds
- 1 teaspoon chia seeds

Instructions

1. Combine oats, dates, and 2½ cups water in a medium bowl. Cover and refrigerate overnight. If using frozen strawberries and raspberries for sauce, thaw fruit in the refrigerator overnight.

2. In the morning, transfer oats mixture to a saucepan. Bring to boiling over medium heat. Cover and simmer 10 minutes or until oats are tender and the water has been cooked off. Remove from heat. Stir in vanilla. Set aside.

3. In a blender combine fresh (or thawed frozen) strawberries and raspberries. Blend into a sauce.

4. To serve, divide oatmeal between two bowls. Top with enough berry sauce to cover oatmeal. Arrange fresh fruit on top. Garnish with almonds and seeds.

7. Quick Brown Rice Congee
Prep-Time: 30 Minutes

Cook Time: 30 minutes

Total Time: 1 hour minutes

Servings: 4

Ingredients

- 1 cup dried brown rice
- 1 14-oz. package extra-firm tofu, drained and cut into cubes
- 8 oz. sliced cremini mushrooms
- 3 cups mushroom or vegetable broth
- 1 tablespoons reduced-sodium soy sauce
- 3 slices fresh ginger root
- 2 cloves garlic, minced (2 tsp.)
- 2 scallions (green onions), thinly sliced
- Sesame seeds, for garnish

Instructions

1. Cook brown rice according to package directions. Set aside.

2. Preheat the oven to 400°F, and line 2 baking sheets with parchment paper or silicone baking mats. Spread tofu cubes on one baking sheet and mushroom slices on the other. Roast 10 minutes. Flip tofu cubes and

mushroom slices, and roast 8 to 10 minutes more or until browned on the edges.

3. Meanwhile, bring the rice, broth, soy sauce, ginger, and garlic to a simmer in a large saucepan. Simmer, partially covered, 10 minutes, or until rice is soft and has absorbed some of the broth. Spoon the congee (rice) into bowls, and top with roasted tofu cubes, mushrooms, sliced green onions, and sesame seeds.

8. Pumpkin Spice Muffins

Prep-Time: 10 Minutes

Cook Time: 40 minutes

Total Time: 50 minutes

Servings: 12

Ingredients

- 1½ cups canned pumpkin
- ¾ cup pitted whole dates
- ¾ cup unsweetened almond milk
- 1 teaspoon vanilla
- 1 tablespoon ground flaxseeds
- 1½ cups whole wheat pastry flour
- ½ cup oat flour
- 2 teaspoons regular or sodium-free baking powder
- 2 teaspoons pumpkin pie spice
- ½ teaspoon baking soda
- ¼ teaspoon sea salt
- 2 tablespoons broken pecans

Instructions

1. Preheat oven to 350°F. If desired, line twelve 2½-inch nonstick muffin cups with silicone cupcake liners.

2. In a medium bowl microwave pumpkin, dates, milk, and vanilla 2½ minutes or until dates are softened; cool slightly. In a small bowl combine flaxseeds and 3 tablespoons warm water. Let stand 5 minutes.

3. Transfer pumpkin mixture to a food processor; cover and process until smooth. Add flaxseed mixture; cover and process 10 seconds more.

4. In a medium bowl stir together the next six ingredients (through salt). Add flour mixture to pumpkin mixture in food processor. Cover and process 10 to 15 seconds or just until moistened. (Batter should be lumpy.

5. Spoon batter into the prepared muffin cups. Top with pecans; press lightly. Bake 30 to 35 minutes or until a toothpick comes out clean. Cool in muffin cups on a wire rack 10 minutes. Remove from muffin cups and silicone liners. Serve warm or cool completely on rack.

9. Mini Apple-Raisin Muffins

Prep-Time: 30 Minutes

Cook Time: 50 minutes

Total Time: 1 hour 20 minutes

Servings: 24

Ingredients

- 1 15-oz. can no-salt-added garbanzo beans (chickpeas)
- ⅔ cup mashed banana
- ½ cup pitted whole dates, snipped (3.5 oz.)
- ¼ cup unsweetened, unflavored plant-based milk
- 2 tablespoons flaxseed meal
- 1 teaspoon orange zest
- 1 tablespoon orange juice
- 1 teaspoon pure vanilla extract
- 2 cups white whole wheat flour
- 1½ teaspoon regular or sodium-free baking powder
- ½ teaspoon ground cinnamon
- ¼ teaspoon fine sea salt
- ½ cup finely chopped apple
- ½ cup raisins, snipped

Instructions

1. Preheat oven to 400°F. Line mini muffin cups with foil liners (do not use paper liners) or use a nonstick

mini muffin pan. Drain garbanzo beans, reserving ½ cup of the liquid (aquafaba). Cover and chill beans up to 3 days for another use.

2. In a blender or food processor combine the ½ cup aquafaba and the next seven ingredients (through vanilla). Cover and blend or process until smooth.

3. In a large bowl stir together flour, baking powder, cinnamon, and sea salt. Add banana mixture all at once to flour mixture. Stir just until moistened (batter should be lumpy). Fold in apple and raisins. Spoon batter into the prepared muffin cups, filling each two-thirds full.

4. Bake 11 to 14 minutes or until a toothpick inserted in a muffin's center comes out clean. Cool in muffin pan on a wire rack 5 minutes. Remove muffins from pan and cool completely.

10. Pumpkin Seed Granola with Millet and Oats

Prep-Time: 15 Minutes

Cook Time: 50 minutes

Total Time: 1 hour 5 minutes

Servings: 6

Ingredients

- ½ cup pitted whole dates
- 2 tablespoons ground flaxseeds
- 2 cups thick-cut or regular rolled oats
- ½ cup sliced almonds
- ¼ cup millet
- 1 tablespoon sesame seeds
- 1 tablespoon ground cinnamon
- 1 teaspoon ground ginger
- ¼ teaspoon sea salt
- ½ cup raw pumpkin seeds (pepitas)
- ½ cup raisins

Instructions

1. Preheat oven to 325°F. In a small bowl combine the dates and ¾ cup warm water. Let stand at least 5 minutes or until softened.

2. In another small bowl combine the flaxseeds and 6 tablespoons warm water. Let stand 5 minutes.

3. In a large bowl combine the next seven ingredients (through salt). Place dates with liquid in a blender. Cover and blend until smooth. Stir pureed dates and flaxseeds with liquid into oat mixture. Spread in a 15x10-inch baking pan.

4. Bake 45 minutes or until golden, stirring every 15 to 20 minutes and adding pumpkin seeds halfway through baking. Cool in pan on a wire rack 10 minutes. Stir in raisins. Store, uncovered, at room temperature up to 10 days or freeze, covered, up to 2 months.

LUNCH

11. Butternut Squash Mac and Cheese with Broccoli

Prep-Time: 30 Minutes

Cook Time: 30 minutes

Total Time: 1 hour

Servings: 6

Ingredients

- 1 medium butternut squash (1¾ lb.)
- 1 onion, finely chopped (1 cup)
- 4 cloves garlic, minced
- ½ teaspoon finely chopped fresh thyme
- 2 cups unsweetened, unflavored plant milk, such as almond, soy, cashew, or rice
- 2 tablespoons nutritional yeast
- 1 tablespoon white wine vinegar
- ¼ tsp. sea salt
- ⅛ tsp. freshly ground black pepper
- 3 cups dried whole grain penne pasta (8 oz.)
- 3 cups small broccoli florets
- Fresh basil leaves

Instructions

1. Peel squash; halve squash and remove seeds. Cut squash into large pieces. Place squash pieces in a steamer basket in a large pan. Add water to saucepan to just below basket. Bring to boiling. Steam, covered, about 12 minutes or until tender.

2. Heat a large saucepan over medium. Add onion, garlic, thyme, and ¼ cup water to pan. Cook about 10 minutes or until onion is tender, stirring occasionally and adding water, 1 to 2 Tbsp. at a time, as needed to prevent sticking.

3. Transfer onion mixture to a blender. Add squash and the next five ingredients (through pepper). Cover and blend until smooth. Pour squash mixture into a large saucepan.

4. Cook pasta according to package directions, adding broccoli the last 5 minutes of cooking; drain. Add drained pasta and broccoli to squash mixture; toss to coat. Serve warm topped with fresh basil.

12. Carrot Dogs

Prep-Time: 20 Minutes

Cook Time: 4 hours 20 minutes

Total Time: 4 hour 40 minutes

Servings: 8

Ingredients

- 8 large carrots
- 1 cup low-sodium vegetable broth
- ¼ cup apple cider vinegar
- 2 tablespoons reduced-sodium soy sauce or tamari
- 2 tablespoons pure maple syrup
- 2 teaspoons smoked paprika
- 2 teaspoons dry mustard
- ½ teaspoon ground coriander
- ½ teaspoon garlic powder
- ½ teaspoon onion powder
- ½ teaspoon liquid smoke
- Dash ground cloves
- 8 whole wheat hot dog buns, toasted if desired
- ½ of a red onion, finely chopped (¼ cup)
- 3 tablespoons stone-ground mustard
- ½ of a medium cucumber, spiralized

Instructions

1. Peel carrots and trim to 6 inches long. Trim wide end to make a consistent thickness. Place carrots in a large saucepan; add water to cover. Cover pan and bring to boiling; reduce heat to low. Cook carrots 8 to 10 minutes, until just tender. Drain well.

2. Place carrots in a large resealable plastic bag set in a shallow dish. For marinade, in a bowl combine the next 11 ingredients (through cloves) and ½ cup water. Pour over carrots; seal bag. Chill 4 to 24 hours, turning occasionally. Drain and discard marinade.

3. Grill carrots, covered, over medium-high 5 to 8 minutes or until grill marks start to appear, turning occasionally. Or place carrots in a foil-lined baking pan and bake at 450°F 8 to 10 minutes or until lightly browned on edges.

4. Place grilled carrots in buns. Top with red onion, mustard, and cucumber.

13. Roasted Cauliflower and Quinoa Casserole

Prep-Time: 20 Minutes

Cook Time: 1 hours 20 minutes

Total Time: 1 hour 40 minutes

Servings: 12 cup

Ingredients

- 2 cups dry quinoa
- 3½ cups vegetable broth, divided
- ½ medium onion, cut into ¼-inch dice (1 cup)
- 6 cloves garlic, minced
- 1 tablespoon Italian seasoning
- 1 medium head cauliflower, cut into 1-inch florets (about 6 cups)
- 1 tablespoon white wine vinegar
- Sea salt and freshly ground black pepper
- 3 cups store-bought marinara sauce
- 1 cup frozen green peas, thawed

Instructions

1. In a large saucepan combine quinoa and 3 cups broth. Bring to a boil; then reduce heat to low and cover pan. Simmer 20 minutes. Remove from heat and let stand 10 minutes. Drain off any excess water, if needed.

2. In a skillet, combine onion, garlic, Italian seasoning, and ¼ cup broth; cook over medium for 10 minutes or until onion is tender, adding more broth, 1 to 2 tablespoons at a time, as needed to prevent sticking. Add cauliflower to skillet and cook 10 to 15 minutes more, or until cauliflower is just starting to get tender. Do not overcook. Add vinegar and season with salt and pepper.

3. Preheat oven to 350°F. Fluff quinoa with a fork; then spread it in an even layer in the bottom of a large casserole dish. Cover quinoa with an even layer of marinara sauce, followed by cauliflower and green peas on top. Bake uncovered 20 to 25 minutes, until there is browning on the cauliflower. Serve warm.

14. Italian-Style Zucchini and Chickpea Sauté

Prep-Time: 25 Minutes

Cook Time: 30 minutes

Total Time: 55 minutes

Servings: 6 cup

Ingredients

- 1 onion, chopped (1 cup)
- 1 large red bell pepper, chopped (1 cup)
- 6 cloves garlic, minced
- 1 teaspoon dried oregano
- ½ teaspoon dried thyme
- 3 medium zucchini, halved lengthwise and cut into ¼-inch slices (4 cups)
- 1 15-oz. can chickpeas, rinsed and drained (1½ cups)
- 1 cup oil-free marinara sauce
- 1 tablespoon white wine vinegar
- Sea salt and freshly ground black pepper, to taste
- 8 to 10 fresh basil leaves, chopped

Instructions

1. Heat an extra-large skillet over medium. Add the first five ingredients (through thyme); cook 10 minutes, stirring often and adding water, 1 to 2 Tbsp. at a time, as needed to prevent sticking.

31

2. Add zucchini; cook 10 minutes more or until zucchini is tender. Stir in chickpeas, marinara sauce, and vinegar. Season with salt and black pepper. Heat through. Serve immediately garnished with basil.

15. Potato and Artichoke Heart Pasta Salad

Prep-Time: 30 Minutes

Cook Time: 30 minutes

Total Time: 1 hour

Servings: 10 cup

Ingredients

- 1½ pounds potatoes, any variety, scrubbed and cut into 1-inch chunks
- 2 cups dry whole grain pasta, any variety
- 1 15-ounce can artichoke hearts, rinsed, drained and quartered lengthwise
- 4 ounces hearts of palm, sliced (½ cup)
- 1 cup cherry tomatoes, cut into halves
- 2 stalks scallions (green onions), thinly sliced
- 2 tablespoons finely chopped fresh dill (or 1 tablespoon dried dill weed)
- 1 12-ounce package silken tofu, drained
- 2½ tablespoons white wine vinegar
- 2 small cloves garlic
- 1½ teaspoons yellow mustard
- Sea salt
- ¼ to ½ cup unsweetened, unflavored plant-based milk

Instructions

1. Place a steamer insert in a saucepan over 1 to 2 inches of water. Bring water to boiling. Add potatoes to basket, cover, and steam for 20 minutes, or until potatoes are very tender when pierced with the tip of a sharp knife. Transfer potatoes to a large bowl to cool.

2. Cook pasta according to package directions; drain. Rinse with cold water; drain again. Transfer to the bowl with the potatoes. Add the artichoke hearts, hearts of palm, tomatoes, scallions, and dill.

3. In a blender, combine the tofu, vinegar, garlic, and mustard. Blend into a smooth sauce. Season to taste with salt and pepper.

4. Add the sauce to the bowl and mix well. Taste and adjust seasoning. Chill in the fridge or serve at room temperature. Note that pasta will absorb the sauce as it sits: Just before serving, add the plant-based milk 1 to 2 Tbsp. at a time, to achieve desired texture and creaminess.

16. Buffalo Cauliflower Pita Pockets

Prep-Time: 30 Minutes

Cook Time: 30 minutes

Total Time: 1 hour

Servings: 8 Pockets

Ingredients

- 2 15-oz. cans no-salt-added chickpeas
- 2 tablespoons white wine vinegar
- 1 tablespoon Dijon mustard
- 1 to 2 tablespoons hot sauce
- 1 tablespoon no-salt-added tomato paste
- 1 12- to 16-oz. package frozen cauliflower, large florets cut into bite-size pieces
- ½ cup chopped onion
- ½ cup chopped carrot
- 3 cloves garlic, minced
- Freshly ground black pepper, to taste
- 8 lettuce leaves
- 4 whole wheat pita bread rounds, halved crosswise and warmed
- ½ cup finely chopped celery
- Lemon wedges

Instructions

1. Drain garbanzo beans, reserving liquid (aquafaba). Rinse beans off. In a medium bowl mash ½ cup of the beans; set remaining beans aside. In a small bowl whisk together ¼ cup of the aquafaba (reserve remaining aquafaba for another use), the vinegar, mustard, hot sauce, and tomato paste. Stir into mashed beans.

2. In an extra-large skillet cook cauliflower, onion, carrot, and garlic over medium 3 to 4 minutes, stirring occasionally and adding water, 1 to 2 Tbsp. at a time, as needed to prevent sticking. Add whole beans and mashed bean mixture. Cook about 5 minutes or until most of the liquid has been absorbed and cauliflower is tender. Season with pepper. Place one lettuce leaf in each pita half, then fill pitas with cauliflower mixture and top with celery. Serve with lemon wedges and, if desired, additional hot sauce.

17. Spring Roll Bowls

Prep-Time: 30 Minutes

Cook Time: 30 minutes

Total Time: 1 hour

Servings: 2 Bowls

Ingredients

Peanut Sauce:

- 2 Tbsp. natural creamy peanut butter
- 1 Tbsp. lime juice
- 1 Tbsp. pure maple syrup
- 1 Tbsp. snipped fresh cilantro
- 1 tsp. grated fresh ginger
- 1 clove garlic, minced
- Sea salt and freshly ground black pepper, to taste

Bowls:

- 4 oz. brown rice noodles
- ⅔ cup frozen edamame
- 1 cup fresh snow peas, halved
- ½ of a medium cucumber, cut into bite-size strips
- ½ cup coarsely shredded carrot
- 2 Tbsp. sliced radishes

Optional Toppings:

- Crushed peanuts

- Sliced Thai or jalapeño peppers
- Sliced green onions
- Snipped fresh cilantro
- Lime wedges

Instructions

1. Make Peanut Sauce: In a small bowl whisk together natural creamy peanut butter, lime juice, pure maple syrup, and snipped fresh cilantro, grated fresh ginger, minced garlic, and, if desired, crushed red pepper. Gradually stir in 2 Tbsp. water until sauce is the consistency of maple syrup. Season to taste with sea salt and freshly ground black pepper.

2. Cook noodles according to package directions. Rinse well with cold water; drain. Cook edamame according to package directions.

3. Divide noodles between two bowls and top with edamame, snow peas, cucumber, carrot, and radishes. Drizzle Peanut Sauce evenly over bowls. Add desired toppings.

18. "Stuffinged" Sweet Potatoes

Prep-Time: 30 Minutes

Cook Time: 1 hour 40 minutes

Total Time: 2 hour 10 minutes

Makes: 8 Stuffed Potato Halves

Ingredients

- 4 large sweet potatoes, scrubbed and patted dry (about 3 lb.)
- 1½ cups chopped fresh cremini mushrooms (4 oz.)
- ½ cup chopped onion
- 2 stalks celery, sliced (½ cup)
- 2 cloves garlic, minced
- 2 15-oz. cans no-salt-added chickpeas, rinsed and drained
- 2 cups ½-inch whole wheat bread cubes, dried
- ½ cup chopped fresh parsley
- 1½ teaspoon poultry seasoning
- Sea salt and freshly ground black pepper, to taste
- ¼ to ⅓ cup low-sodium vegetable broth

Instructions

1. Preheat oven to 400°F. Prick sweet potatoes all over with a fork. Place in a 3-qt. rectangular baking dish. Bake about 45 minutes or until just tender when

pierced with a knife. Let stand until cool enough to handle.

2. Meanwhile, for stuffing, in a large nonstick skillet cook mushrooms, onion, celery, and garlic over medium 5 minutes, stirring occasionally and adding water, 1 to 2 Tbsp. at a time, as needed to prevent sticking.

3. In a food processor combine mushroom mixture and chickpeas; pulse until chopped. Transfer to a bowl. Add bread cubes, parsley, poultry seasoning, salt, and pepper. Drizzle with broth, tossing just until moistened.

4. Cut sweet potatoes in half lengthwise. Using a sharp knife, score around potato flesh, leaving a ¼-inch shell and being careful not to cut through skin. Score in a crisscross to make ½-inch cubes. Gently scoop cubes out with a spoon. If necessary, cut any large pieces in half to make smaller cubes. Add cubes to stuffing mixture in bowl; gently fold to combine.

5. Arrange potato skin shells in the baking dish. Spoon stuffing into shells. Bake, uncovered, about 20 minutes or until browned and heated through. To transport, place baking dish in an insulated carrier with a hot pack.

19. Roasted Veggie Flatbreads

Prep-Time: 30 Minutes

Cook Time: 45 minutes

Total Time: 1 hour 15 minutes

Makes: 4 Flatbreads

Ingredients

Cornmeal, for dusting:

- 1 recipe Homemade Oil Free Pizza Dough
- 6 baby potatoes, quartered
- 8 Brussels sprouts, quartered
- 1 medium carrot, coarsely chopped
- 1 medium shallot, coarsely chopped
- 1 tablespoon red wine vinegar
- Sea salt and freshly ground black pepper, to taste
- ⅓ cup balsamic vinegar
- 1 cup no-salt-added canned cannellini beans, rinsed and drained
- 1 teaspoon finely chopped fresh sage or ¼ tsp. dried sage, crushed
- 2 cups fresh microgreens

Instructions

1. Preheat oven to 400°F. Lightly sprinkle a large baking sheet with cornmeal.

2. Divide dough into four portions. On a lightly floured surface, roll portions into 7- to 8-inch circles or 10×5-inch ovals. Transfer flatbreads to prepared pan. Bake 10 to 13 minutes or until lightly browned and set (flatbreads may puff). Let cool.

3. Preheat oven to 425°F. Line a 15×10-inch baking pan with foil. Arrange potatoes, Brussels sprouts, carrot, and shallot in prepared baking pan. Sprinkle with red wine vinegar and season with salt and pepper. Roast about 20 minutes or until tender and lightly browned.

4. Meanwhile, for balsamic glaze, in a small saucepan bring balsamic vinegar to boiling; reduce heat. Simmer, uncovered, about 6 minutes or until mixture has reduced to about 1 ½ Tbsp. and thickened to a syrup consistency.

5. In a bowl mash beans with a fork and stir in sage and 2 tsp. water. Spread on flatbreads. Top with roasted vegetables. Remove foil from baking sheet; transfer flatbreads to baking sheet. Bake 5 minutes to heat through.

6. Drizzle flatbreads with balsamic glaze and top with microgreens.

20. Blueberry Spinach Salad Bowl with Orange Vinaigrette

Prep-Time: 15 Minutes

Cook Time: 30 minutes

Total Time: 45 minutes

Makes: 2 Bowls

Ingredients

Orange Vinaigrette:

- ½ tsp. orange zest
- 2 tablespoons juice from 1 orange
- 1 tablespoon white wine vinegar
- 1 tablespoon snipped fresh herbs, such as parsley, chives, or dill
- 1½ teaspoon Dijon-style mustard
- Sea salt and freshly ground black pepper, to taste

Bowls:

- 1 small sweet potato, peeled and thinly sliced
- 1 teaspoon orange juice
- ⅛ teaspoon curry powder
- ⅛ teaspoon paprika
- 3 cups fresh baby spinach
- 1¼ cups cooked wheat berries
- ½ of a 15-oz. can no-salt-added cannellini beans, rinsed and drained

- ⅔ cup fresh blueberries
- ½ of an avocado, seeded, peeled, and sliced
- Optional toppings: sliced green onions, sliced radishes, and/or fresh orange slices

Instructions

1. Make Orange Vinaigrette: Remove ½ tsp. zest and squeeze 2 Tbsp. juice from 1 orange. In a small bowl whisk together zest and juice, white wine vinegar, fresh herbs, and Dijon-style mustard. Season with salt and pepper to taste. Set aside.

2. Preheat oven to 375°F. Line a baking sheet with parchment paper. Arrange sweet potato slices in a single layer on baking sheet. In a small bowl stir together orange juice, curry powder, and paprika. Brush over sweet potato. Bake 15 to 20 minutes or until tender. Cool potato in pan on a wire rack.

3. Divide spinach between two bowls. Top with sweet potato, wheat berries, beans, blueberries, and avocado. Drizzle Orange Vinaigrette evenly over bowls. Add desired toppings.

DINNER

21. Lemon Broccoli Rotini

Prep-Time: 30 Minutes

Cook Time: 30 minutes

Total Time: 1 hour

Makes: 12 Cups

Ingredients

- 3 cups sliced cremini mushrooms (8 oz.)
- 1 medium onion, chopped (1 cup)
- 4 cloves garlic, minced
- 4 cups dried whole wheat rotini pasta (12 oz.)
- 2 cups low-sodium vegetable broth
- 2 cups unsweetened, unflavored plant-based milk
- 1 lemon
- 1 16-oz. package frozen broccoli florets (or 6 cups fresh)
- ½ cup chopped roasted red bell peppers
- 1 teaspoon chopped fresh tarragon
- Sea salt and freshly ground black pepper, to taste

Instructions

1. In a large saucepan cook mushrooms, onion, and garlic over medium 2 to 3 minutes, stirring occasionally and adding water, 1 to 2 Tbsp. at a time, as needed to prevent sticking. Stir in rotini, vegetable broth, and milk. Bring to boiling; reduce heat. Cover and simmer 5 to 7 minutes or until pasta is nearly tender.

2. Remove 1 tsp. zest from lemon and stir into saucepan with pasta. Stir in broccoli, red peppers, and tarragon. Cook about 5 minutes or until broccoli and pasta are tender. Stir in 1 Tbsp. of juice from lemon. Season with salt and black pepper. If desired, sprinkle with additional lemon zest and serve with lemon wedges.

22. Garlicky Bok Choy Noodle Soup

Prep-Time: 35 Minutes

Cook Time: 40 minutes

Total Time: 1 hour 15 minutes

Makes: About 11½ Cups

Ingredients

- 4 cups no-salt-added vegetable broth
- 4 cloves garlic, minced
- 1 tablespoons minced fresh ginger
- 2 teaspoons reduced-sodium soy sauce
- 6 ounces dried brown rice pad Thai noodles
- 12 baby carrots with green tops, halved lengthwise, or 2 cups bias-sliced carrots
- 3 ounces extra-firm light silken-style tofu, cut into ¼-inch cubes
- 2 heads baby bok choy, halved lengthwise
- 12 thin spears asparagus, trimmed
- 1 cup fresh shiitake mushrooms, stems removed, or oyster mushrooms, sliced
- 4 scallions (green onions), green tops trimmed and cut in half lengthwise
- 1 lime, cut into wedges

Instructions

1. In a 5- to 6-qt. Dutch oven combine 4 cups water, the broth, garlic, ginger, and soy sauce. Bring to boiling; reduce heat. Cover and simmer 10 minutes to allow flavors to meld.

2. Add noodles, carrots, and tofu. Simmer, uncovered, 8 minutes, stirring occasionally. Add bok choy, asparagus, mushrooms, and scallions. Simmer, uncovered, 1 minute more. Serve in shallow bowls with lime wedges.

23. Spicy Tomato Sushi Rolls

Prep-Time: 1 hour

Cook Time: 1 hour

Total Time: 2 hour

Makes: 4 Rolls

Ingredients

- 1½ cups low-sodium vegetable broth
- ¾ cup dry short grain brown rice
- 1½ cups frozen riced butternut squash
- 4 roma tomatoes, seeded and chopped (2 cups)
- 1 tablespoon reduced-sodium tamari
- 1 teaspoon grated fresh ginger
- 1 tablespoon sriracha sauce
- 2 teaspoons tahini
- 2 tablespoons brown rice vinegar
- 1 tablespoon pure maple syrup
- 4 8-inch toasted nori sheets
- ½ of a medium avocado, peeled and sliced
- 1 Persian cucumber, seeded and cut lengthwise into ¼-inch strips (5½ oz.)
- 2 carrots, coarsely shredded (1 cup)
- 4 scallions (green onions), trimmed to 6 inches and cut lengthwise into strips

Instructions

1. In a small saucepan bring broth to boiling. Add rice; reduce heat. Cover and simmer about 40 minutes or until liquid is absorbed. Stir in frozen riced butternut squash. Let stand 5 minutes.

2. Meanwhile, for spicy tomatoes, in a bowl stir together the next five ingredients (through tahini).

3. Stir rice vinegar and maple syrup into brown rice mixture.

4. Lay a sushi mat on a cutting board; place a nori sheet lengthwise on mat. With damp fingers, spread one-fourth of the rice mixture over bottom two-thirds of the nori, leaving a ¼-inch border on side edges. Arrange one fourth of the avocado, cucumber, carrots, tomato mixture, and scallions along center of rice layer. Roll up nori toward the unfilled edge, using sushi mat to lift and tightly roll. Brush unfilled edge with water and press over top of roll. Repeat with remaining ingredients, making four rolls total. Slice each roll into 1-inch slices to serve.

24. Vegan Welsh Rarebit with Mushrooms

Prep-Time: 25 minutes

Cook Time: 30 minutes

Total Time: 55 minutes

Makes: 8 Tartines

Ingredients

- 1 8-oz. pkg. sliced fresh button or cremini mushrooms
- 1 onion, thinly sliced (1 cup)
- ¼ teaspoon dried thyme, crushed
- 1 15-oz. can Great Northern beans, rinsed and drained (1½ cups cooked)
- 2 tablespoons Dijon-style or English mustard
- 2 tablespoons nutritional yeast
- 2 tablespoons cashew butter or almond butter
- Sea salt and freshly ground black pepper, to taste
- 4 sprouted whole grain English muffins, split and toasted
- Paprika
- Chopped fresh parsley

Instructions

1. In a large skillet combine mushrooms, onion, thyme, and 1 cup water. Cover and bring to a simmer over medium. Simmer 10 minutes or until mushrooms and

onion slices are tender. Uncover and cook 1 to 2 minutes more or until most of the liquid has evaporated.

2. Meanwhile, in a blender combine the next four ingredients (through nut butter) and ½ cup hot water. Cover and blend to a smooth sauce.

3. Stir sauce into mushroom mixture. Simmer 1 to 2 minutes or until thickened. Season with salt and pepper.

4. Preheat broiler. To assemble, place toasted English muffins on a baking sheet. Top with mushroom mixture. Broil 4 to 5 inches from heat 4 to 5 minutes or until lightly browned on top. Sprinkle with paprika and parsley.

25. Chickpea and Potato–Stuffed Poblano Peppers

Prep-Time: 40 minutes

Cook Time: 1 hour

Total Time: 1 hour 40 minutes

Makes: 4 Stuffed Peppers

Ingredients

- 4 oz. cremini mushrooms, sliced (1½ cups)
- 2 to 3 teaspoons ground turmeric
- 1 tsp. ground cumin
- 2 cloves garlic, minced
- ¼ teaspoon ground coriander
- ⅛ teaspoon cayenne pepper
- 1 15-oz. can no-salt-added garbanzo beans (chickpeas), rinsed and drained
- ¼ cup toasted almonds
- 2 cups chopped yellow potatoes (about 12 oz.)
- 1 small onion, chopped (½ cup)
- ¼ cup chopped fresh cilantro
- Sea salt and freshly ground black pepper, to taste
- 4 large fresh poblano chile peppers
- 1 lime, cut into wedges
- Fresh cilantro, for garnish (optional)

Instructions

1. For chickpea sausage, in an extra-large skillet cook mushrooms over medium-high 6 to 8 minutes or until lightly browned and tender, stirring occasionally and adding water, 1 to 2 Tbsp. at a time, as needed to prevent sticking.

2. In a large bowl combine the next five ingredients (through cayenne). In a food processor combine mushrooms, chickpeas, almonds, and 1 Tbsp. water. Pulse until chopped. Add mixture to seasonings in bowl; stir to combine.

3. Place potatoes and onion in a steamer basket set in the extra-large skillet. Add water to just below basket. Bring to boiling. Steam, covered, 12 to 14 minutes or until tender. Add steamed potatoes and onion to mixture in bowl. Toss to combine. Stir in cilantro. Season with salt and black pepper.

4. Make a lengthwise slit down one side of each poblano pepper. Carefully remove seeds and membranes with a small spoon, and rinse out any remaining seeds with water. Spoon chickpea sausage into peppers.

5. Place filled peppers in the steamer basket in the skillet. If necessary, add water to just below basket. Bring to boiling. Steam, covered, 20 minutes or until peppers are crisp-tender and filling is heated through. Serve with lime wedges. If desired, top with additional cilantro.

26. Peach-Corn Salsa with Chili-Lime Chips

Prep-Time: 30 minutes

Cook Time: 2 hour 30 minutes

Total Time: 3 hour

Makes: 6 Cups

Ingredients

- 2 ears sweet corn, husks and silks removed
- 5 tablespoons lime juice
- 1 fresh poblano chile pepper, halved and seeded
- 1 small yellow onion, cut crosswise into ½-inch slices
- 1 medium peach, halved and pitted
- 1 15-oz. can black-eyed peas, rinsed and drained
- 2 tomatoes, seeded and chopped (1 cup)
- ¼ cup chopped fresh cilantro
- ¼ teaspoon ground cumin
- Sea salt and freshly ground black pepper, to taste
- 12 corn tortillas
- Chili powder, to taste

Instructions

1. Cook corn in enough boiling water to cover 3 minutes; drain. Meanwhile, combine 1 Tbsp. lime juice with 1 Tbsp. water. Brush corn, poblano, onion slices, and peach halves with lime juice mixture. Grill, uncovered,

over medium-high about 10 minutes or until tender and slightly charred, turning as needed and brushing with additional lime juice mixture to prevent drying. Transfer to a cutting board; let cool. Chop poblano, onion, and peach. Cut corn from cobs.

2. In a large bowl combine 3 Tbsp. lime juice, the corn, poblano, onion, peach, and the next four ingredients (through cumin). Season with salt and black pepper. Cover and chill 2 hours before serving.

3. To make Chili-Lime Chips: Preheat oven to 375°F. Brush both sides of 12 corn tortillas lightly with 1 Tbsp. lime juice. Sprinkle both sides with freshly ground black pepper and chili powder to taste. Cut each tortilla into six wedges. Arrange pieces in a single layer on large baking sheets. Bake 18 to 22 minutes or until crisp and edges are golden brown.

4. Store Peach Caviar in the refrigerator and cooled Chili-Lime Chips Chips in an airtight container up to 3 days.

27. Vegan Chili Cheese Fries

Prep-Time: 1 hour

Cook Time: 1 hour 30 minutes

Total Time: 2 hour 30 minutes

Ingredients

Fries And Cheesy Sauce:

- 4 pounds Russet potatoes, cut into ½-inch-thick wedges
- 1 cup unsweetened, unflavored plant-based milk
- ¼ cup nutritional yeast
- 1 tablespoon lemon juice
- 1 teaspoon garlic powder
- Sea salt and freshly ground black pepper, to taste

Chili And Garnishes:

- 1 medium onion, cut into ¼-inch dice (about 2 cups)
- 6 cloves garlic, minced
- 2 15-ounce cans red kidney beans, drained and rinsed (3 cups)
- 1 15-ounce can fire-roasted tomatoes (1½ cups)
- 4 tablespoons mild (or hot) chili seasoning
- 2 tablespoons lemon juice
- Sea salt and freshly ground black pepper
- 2 stalks scallions, thinly sliced (¼ cup)
- 2 tablespoons chopped fresh cilantro

Instructions

1. Preheat oven to 400°F.

2. Place potato wedges in a steamer basket in a saucepan. Add water to saucepan to just below basket. Cover pan and steam potatoes 15 to 20 minutes or until tender. Transfer ¼ of the potatoes to a bowl and set aside. Spread out the remaining potatoes in a 13x9-inch casserole dish; bake 20 minutes until fries are crispy and brown.

3. For Cheesy Sauce, add milk, nutritional yeast, lemon juice, and garlic powder to bowl with reserved steamed potatoes. Mix well, using a potato masher to mash the potatoes into a smooth sauce. Season with salt and pepper.

4. For chili, in a sauté pan, combine onion and garlic with ¼ cup of water. Sauté 10 minutes on medium heat until onion is tender, adding water, 1 to 2 tablespoons at a time, as needed to prevent sticking. Add beans, tomatoes, and chili seasoning, and cook 5 minutes more or until chili thickens. Add lemon juice, and season with salt and pepper.

5. To assemble Chili Cheese Fries, spread chili over baked fries in casserole dish. Dollop Cheesy Sauce over chili layer. Bake 20 minutes or until Cheesy Sauce is lightly browned.

6. Remove from oven and garnish with scallions and cilantro. Serve immediately.

28. Tex-Mex Potato Skins

Prep-Time: 30 minutes

Cook Time: 1 hour 30 minutes

Total Time: 2 hour

Makes: 16 Potato Skins

Ingredients

- 8 small (4- to 6-ounce) potatoes, scrubbed
- 1 (15-ounce) can black beans, rinsed and drained (1½ cups)
- 1 cup fresh or frozen corn, thawed
- ½ teaspoon ground cumin
- ½ teaspoon garlic powder
- ¼ teaspoon chipotle powder
- ½ teaspoon sea salt, divided
- 2 tablespoons lemon juice, divided
- 1 cup unsweetened, unflavored plant milk
- ¼ cup nutritional yeast
- 1 teaspoon onion powder
- 1 cup store-bought pico de gallo
- ¼ cup thinly sliced scallions

Instructions

1. Preheat oven to 450°F. Scrub potatoes and use a fork to poke several holes in each one. Arrange potatoes on

a baking sheet and bake 40 to 60 minutes or until tender when pierced with a fork. Cool on baking sheet.

2. Slice potatoes in half lengthwise. Carefully scoop out and reserve most of the potato flesh, leaving a thin layer of potato flesh with the skin to help retain the potato's shape.

3. To make the filling, in a medium bowl, combine 2 cups of potato flesh, black beans, corn, cumin, garlic powder, chipotle powder, ¼ teaspoon of salt, and 1 tablespoon lemon juice. Mix well. Set aside.

4. To make cheese sauce, place 1 cup of potato flesh in a blender. Add milk, nutritional yeast, remaining 1 tablespoon lemon juice, the onion powder, pepper, and remaining ¼ teaspoon salt. Blend mixture to a smooth, thick sauce, adding water a little at a time if needed to reach a thick saucy consistency.

5. Roughly 30 minutes before desired serving time, preheat the oven to 375°F. Fill each potato skin with the filling mixture; then drizzle 1 tablespoon sauce over each filled potato. Bake on the oven's top rack for 10 to 20 minutes, or until sauce and edges of potatoes are just starting to brown.

6. Remove stuffed potatoes from oven and top with pico de gallo and scallions. Serve immediately.

29. Vegan Nachos Verdes

Prep-Time: 1 hour

Cook Time: 1 hour 30 minutes

Total Time: 2 hour 30 minutes

Makes: 10 Cups

Ingredients

Tortilla Chips:

- 12 oil-free corn tortillas, cut into 1½ inch pieces (about 3 cups)

Zesty Beans:

- 1½ cups frozen lima beans, thawed
- 1½ cups frozen corn, thawed
- 1 small onion, cut into ¼-inch dice (1 cup)
- 1 teaspoon minced garlic
- ½ teaspoon ground cumin
- ½ teaspoon dried Mexican oregano
- Sea salt

Green Tofu Sour Cream:

- 1 (12-ounce) package extra-firm tofu
- ¼ cup fresh spinach
- 2 tablespoons lemon juice
- 1 tablespoon white wine vinegar
- ½ teaspoon sea salt

- ¼ teaspoon yellow mustard

Toppings:

- 1 cup store-bought salsa verde
- 4 scallions, thinly sliced (½ cup)
- ¼ cup finely chopped cilantro
- 2 cups romaine lettuce
- 1 avocado, diced
- 1 jalapeño, thinly sliced (optional)

Instructions

1. Preheat the oven to 350°F. Line 2 baking sheets with parchment paper.

2. Spread the tortilla pieces on the baking sheets, and bake for 20 to 25 minutes, or until crisp. Remove from oven and set aside to cool for a few minutes. Leave oven on.

3. Combine the lima beans, corn, onion, garlic, cumin, and oregano in a saute pan with ½ cup of water. Cover pan and cook for 10 minutes, until the beans are tender. Add salt to taste.

4. To make the tofu sour cream, combine the tofu, spinach, lemon juice, vinegar, salt, and mustard in a blender; blend to a smooth paste.

5. Arrange half of the baked tortilla chips in the bottom of a 9x13-inch baking dish. Spread half of the beans mixture over the chips. Dollop one-third of the tofu sour cream and salsa over the top, then sprinkle with half of the scallions and cilantro. Repeat with a second

layer of chips, beans, tofu sour cream, salsa, scallions, and cilantro.

6. Bake for 20 minutes, or until heated through.

7. Remove nachos from oven, and top with remaining salsa and tofu sour cream, plus lettuce, avocado, and jalapeño (if using).

8. Serve immediately.

30. Rustic Bread Bowl with Sun-Dried Tomato and Asparagus Dip

Prep-Time: 1 hour 15 minutes

Cook Time: 1 hour 30 minutes

Total Time: 2 hour 45 minutes

Makes: 1 Loaf And 3 Cups Dip

Ingredients

Bread Bowl:

- 1¼ cups unsweetened plant-based milk, divided
- 1 cup steamed and mashed potatoes (about 1 pound)
- 3 tablespoons lemon juice
- 1½ cups all-purpose flour, plus more for dusting
- 1 cup whole wheat flour
- 1 tablespoon sodium-free baking powder
- ½ teaspoon sodium-free baking soda
- 1 teaspoon sea salt
- 1 pinch ground black pepper
- ½ tablespoon sesame seeds

Dip:

- 10–12 asparagus stalks, trimmed
- 1½ cups unsweetened, unflavored plant-based milk
- ⅓ cup whole wheat flour
- 1 tablespoon red wine vinegar
- 1 tablespoon nutritional yeast

- 2 teaspoons finely chopped fresh rosemary
- ½ tablespoon garlic powder
- ½ tablespoon onion powder
- 4 pieces sun-dried tomatoes
- 1 (14-ounce) can hearts of palm, drained and rinsed
- Sea salt and freshly ground black pepper

Instructions

1. To make Bread Bowl, preheat oven to 375°F. Line a baking sheet with parchment paper.
2. In a mixing bowl combine 1 cup milk, mashed potatoes, and lemon juice. Mix well.
3. In a separate bowl, combine the flours, baking powder, baking soda, salt, and pepper. Mix well.
4. Add the wet ingredients to the dry ingredients; mix gently to combine, but do not knead. Shape the dough into a ball, then flatten it into a large disk that is 1½ inch high and 7 inches in diameter. Press into the middle of the disk to create a well. Line this well with a piece of parchment paper, and fill it with pie weight or dry beans.
5. Brush the surface of the loaf with the remaining ¼ cup milk, and sprinkle with sesame seeds.
6. Bake 50 to 60 minutes until brown on top.
7. Remove bread bowl from the oven and remove the weights. Use a serrated knife to cut wedge-shaped slices into the bread bowl for easier serving, but don't cut all the way through to the bottom.
8. To make Dip, place the asparagus and ¼ cup of water in a skillet; cook for 5 to 7 minutes until cooked but still crunchy; do not overcook. Cool the asparagus under cold running water, and chop into ¼-inch pieces.
9. In a saucepan, mix together the milk, flour, vinegar, nutritional yeast, rosemary, garlic powder, and onion powder. Bring mixture to a boil over medium heat, then reduce heat and simmer for 5 to 7 minutes until

the sauce thickens. Let the sauce cool down for 10 minutes.

10. In the bowl of a food processor, pulse the sun-dried tomatoes to a coarse texture. Add hearts of palm and cooled sauce, then process into a creamy texture.

11. Fold the asparagus into the dip, and season to taste with salt and pepper. Spoon dip into bread bowl just before serving.